NO MORE DIETS

How To Overcome Compulsive Eating, Food Addiction And Emotional Eating For Life

Vivian Weissman

No More Diets: How To Overcome Compulsive Eating, Food Addiction and Emotional Eating For Life

Testimonials

"The power of environment says to be the same because one of our humans needs is to have love and connection. Consciously you don't associate food with emotions. Once you replace the emotional addictiveness and detach from the meaning, your intuition tells you what the body needs. That is what Vivian Weissman is teaching in her programs. For instance, buying organic foods costs a lot cheaper than buying cooked foods. I've replaced my habits with healthy ones and I've lost 38 pounds in six weeks. My diabetes II is virtually gone."
 - *Kal Malik, Author & Speaker* http://kal-malik.com

"During my research on personal development, I have been trying to understand the mindset and outlook that is common in successful people. It was a delight when I have met Vivian Weissman. Her insights have pointed me to some valuable resources on life success. I would recommend her to anyone who wishes to improve their career and life."
 - *Andrea Bizzotti, Acceleration Architect*

"Since I have been implementing these strategies to better my health, I have lost six pounds in one week. I am confident to say that this is something anyone can do."
- *James Yearwood, Super Attendant, Father*

"This book really helped motivate me to take control of my eating. I highly recommend it to anyone wanting to kick start a lifestyle change!"
- *Stacy Clendenen, Writer*

"So glad that I have met Vivian Weissman. She is AMAZING! Where were you 5 years ago? I am kicking carbs, sugar and junk food to the curb."
- *Carmela Chiaramonte, Optician*

"After reading No More Diets all I can say is, 'wow!' What a breath of fresh air to finally find a book that tells it how it really is. I have always been an avid believer that you are what you eat, and your inner thoughts create your outer life. No More Diets confirms the fact that if you don't have the right frame of mind you will fail at any diet or eating plan. For anyone who is serious about their fitness and have had enough of being on a diet every day they should read this book."
- *Judy Robertson*

"My weight has been in a state of fluctuation my entire life as I chased every new fad diet that hit the market. I've tried them all. After reading this book, I'm realizing how wrong my approach to losing weight was. This book was refreshing because Vivian Weissman emphasizes that in order to change, your habits you need to change, your mindset and quit aiming for the quick fix.

The message of No More Diets can be summed up with my favorite quote from the book "Let me tell you a secret about success. You will never have it if you are not willing to pay the price for the promise."

That is such an inspiring message. Between Vivian Weissman's real life anecdotes and the emphasis on food being what nourishes and heals your body this book is truly motivational and I highly recommend it to anyone trying to break free from a food addiction and the perils of yo-yo dieting."
- *Nichole Rogers*

Table Of Contents

Introduction

I want to thank you and congratulate you for downloading this book, *No More Diets: How To Overcome Compulsive Eating, Food Addiction and Emotional Eating For Life.*

In my first publication, I have given you my proven strategy to shedding those unwanted pounds and getting back into those skinny jeans. Even though I am fully endorsing the idea of raw foods, as a life transformation success coach and a former fitness trainer, I have found a few flaws in the system.

In this publication, I would be including the first printing of *30 Days on Raw Foods: How To Stop Self Sabotaging Your Diet Now,* as a guideline for anyone who wants to experience juicing and alkalizing the body. However, this won't be the main focus of this edition.

In the second edition of *No More Diets: How To Overcome Compulsive Eating, Food Addiction and Emotional Eating For Life*, I am going to point out to you what were those flaws and why in the long term, the raw food diet is unconventional for the everyday man or woman who wants to stay fit and healthy.

Back in 2010 I have shared with many of you how I have dropped thirty pounds in thirty days and now kept it off for three years. In this edition of, *No More Diets: How To Overcome Compulsive Eating, Food Addiction & Emotional Eating For Life*, we are still going to incorporate the raw food diet with a more affordable and realistic slant.

This is something anyone who has a desire for change can do and is coachable throughout the process. What I am going to teach you absolutely works and we have seen thousands of testimonials that show how easy it is to virtually experience a total body transformation and potentially add ten to fifteen years to your life in an enjoyable way.

Moreover, this second edition goes into depth about how psychology, physiology and philosophy all ties into nutrition.

Thanks again for downloading this book. I hope you enjoy it.

Chapter One

In this book I have included the first publication of my fitness series: **_30 Days On Raw Foods: How To Stop Self Sabotaging Your Diet Now._**

What you hold in front of you is more than a ten-year study and a philosophy that changed the way people look at their health and wellbeing. The reading of these principles won't do you any good, nor applying some of the teachings in this book.

To obtain the results that you seek, you must take action and apply all that is told to you. I repeat that again since many of the critics that I get online is that my principles are not sound. You can read all you want, but if you do not apply yourself, you will never experience the result that you are looking for. To get the desired results that you seek, you have to take action.

That is the truth. Action, especially massive continuous action will move you from where you are to where you want to be. Consistency is the key. If you want long term results, you have to be consistent and continue taking massive action. Eating healthy one day won't get you to your goal, but staying on target with your goals will. Take what you will in this book. Find what works for you.

My personal journey started at a very young age. Later in my fitness career due to stress I have manifested liver disease and found out that if I didn't make any necessary changes, I wouldn't make it past my eighteenth birthday.

The search for holistic healing led me here, to teaching you my personal philosophy of health and wellness and what I have done that helped me save my own life. Work the plan and it will work for you. Remember, you are in control of your own destiny and circumstances. Nothing changes unless you make a decision to change. It all starts with you.

No matter where you are, take the first actionable step and you will succeed.

In this introductory part of this book, I am going to be very frank with you. I wish to convey truth and honesty about how you can go from where you are to where you want to go with a new vision for life. I will be 100% transparent and show you what works.

What you are about to read may seem harsh and ruthless from your perspective, but my mission here is to help you. A lot of times we hear advice from people and it is sugar coated. I mean, how many times have you found an expert in a particular field or someone who has what you want and all that you hear from them is some motivational pump up. Trust me. This is not going to be a pump up and some rah-rah-you-can-do-it-stuff?

This is not why I am here to do and it is not my personality. I tell you how it is, like it is and present you with the evidence to make up your own mind. So here goes.

Every single success or failure in your life will be the cause of a decision or a lack of one. Everything that you do or don't do is a decision. Picking up this book and reading it was a decision set into action. About a year ago, I met a woman who changed my paradigm of how I view life. Here is what she had said,

"You are just one decision away from having everything that you have ever dreamed of."—Deena Morton.

We are truly just one decision away from having everything that our hearts desire but the sad truth is that most people are not willing to stake their life on it.

A decision to ninety-five percent of the population is just like making a wish list and hoping it will come true. What fails them is not really making a serious attempt to go after what they really want.

They believe that there is some kind of magic fairy flying around granting those wishes by the Law Of Attraction. Understand this—there is no such a thing as the Law Of Attraction. You can't expect to sit down on a fluffy purple pillow with your bathrobe facing the mirror and smiling, saying,

"Everything is going to be okay. My finances are not where they are and my health is not where I want it to be but I know that the Universe is out there and it will support me. The law of attraction is working as I sit on my pillow to meditate and do nothing. I have read all the books and I think I've got it. Think positive. Repeat silly affirmations that I don't believe in and it will happen for me."

If you do that, life is just going to pass you by. So many times have I heard people say that they are going to pray about it and they are waiting for a sign and for their environment to change. Get this straight.

Your life is not going to change until you DECIDE. I am going to ask you to make some serious decisions on your part as you read this book. No messing around and no waiting for next year. This is your time. This is where the buck stops and you ask yourself where you want to go from here. When you make an irrevocable decision, action always flows from it. If you have not made a decision, procrastination and a flock of excuses will take over instead. Make a choice today that this is going to be your year.

Make a choice today that today is going to change and that no matter what circumstances are standing in your way. You are going to find a way to get around them. Remember, decisions are what bring people to the top and a lack of them keeps people where they are.

For the critics out there that I have seen just like this Amazon review post, here is my public response.

"It is simple book for those who don't like to read extensive novels . I wouldn't suggest it for some real problem solving."

All I have to say is that this book is designed for those who want to break free from mediocrity. This book is not going to lay out a plan for you like you see in school or how most people suggest. You have to read between the lines. You have to use your brain and think for yourself.

I am not going to give you all the answers here. Look for ways that this book can help you and help you move toward your goals. It is in the application of this book that you may find results that work for you.

Clearly this person who has left this review on Amazon possibly believes in instant gratification and a magic pill to solve their problems. Whatever the case may be, instant gratification are for sissies. It is for those who want the easy way out and not put in the work.

No More Diets is about understanding why food addictions accumulate and how you can change your behavior if you choose to. Compulsive eating disorders work in the same way. There is a reason why someone reaches for food and why they have set that as a standard for themselves.

Listen, I have been on the other side too. I know how you feel. I've felt the same way and I have looked for ways where I can just get the answer. What is that magic word or magic behavior that I can do where I can still be happy and lose weight? What I have found in my discovery over the years is that if you are waiting for someone to tell you what that is, you are going to be waiting a long time.

Workouts have the word "work" in them for a reason and suggests that a given amount of effort is required on your part. There are people out there that are going to read half way through this book and think that there are no "real solutions" out there for them.

As in the revision of this book takes place, I am trained in sports nutrition and at the same time I am prepping for my very first fitness competition. I tell you this not to impress you, but to impress upon you that anything that you want out of life you have to work for. A sculpted body doesn't just happen overnight and neither does changing your habits. Relearning that diets do not work takes time as well and understanding that the old ways of thinking no longer work.

You need to build a new model so that you can go to the next level. That is what I am doing right now and what I am preparing myself for.

So to give feedback on the reviewer who left a comment about my book on Amazon, maybe this book is not for you. There are tons of information out there on the internet that can give you the solution you are looking for. All I know is that I have tried the conventional ways of thinking at one point and found that you cannot get lasting results. You have to do something different and sometimes it doesn't come in a one, two, three step by step guide like we have been programmed to believe.

If I can summarize this book in any way that I can, you have to think outside the box. You have to expand your thinking. Go beyond what is reasonable and do things that other people think are crazy. Be different. So for those who are still with me and are continuously reading I applaud you. Cheers to the ones who refuse to settle and listen to the critics out there.

Now back to the first publication.

In this book I am going to go over how the food choices that you make today are just a reflection of the habits that you have picked up from authority figures and what happens if you do not change your habits. I am also going to share with you some of my health philosophy and how I got to this point in my life. There will be assignments that you need to do and it will determine whether you succeed or fail. The testimonials that you have read in the beginning of this book were from people who made a decision to take action and better their lives. If it can work for them, it can work for you too.

They wanted to transform their lives and they sought out the information from people and experts who have the know-how to help them. Sure this book is about raw food and how people can virtually and potentially drop ten, twenty, or even thirty pounds, but throughout my ten year study of health and nutrition, I have found that food is just a small fraction of the equation.

Make sure that you are ready mentally as you are physically to make the necessary changes because when you do, it will be a game changer for you and you will not want to go back to the way you have lived before. If you can master your inner world, you can have virtually anything that you want in life. That is not only a promise from me, but social proof from my mentors and master mind groups. Everything that you have in your physical world right now was first a thought.

Thoughts dictate what actions you will take. Learn to take control of your mind and then you will know how to control the body.

"If you are going to doubt something, doubt your limits."—Price Pritchett.

What does it mean to you to suspend disbelief and doubt your limits? Have you ever thought about not believing in anything and having a go at everything? Think about it, how would life look like for you?

From a very young age, we have been taught that there are certain things in life that we can't do and there are certain things that are not possible.

Those belief systems have formed out self-image and how we view the world today. So if I were to tell you that raw foods can help you restore your body and you were taught that it is all about genetics, we would have a very interesting debate. I can tell you that you do not have to believe a word that I say. Try it out for yourself. For thirty-days I want you to suspend disbelief that you can achieve results on the raw food diet, but here is the catch—you have to do what is instructed in this book to win.

Chapter Two

Never let anyone tell you that you can't do something. When you let others pollute your mind and tell you that it can't be done, you can only think two ways.

The first is,"*I am just that much closer to what I want in life*" and the other is, *"they are right."* Which one will you pick?

You see, when I was born at twenty-four weeks and the doctors told my parents that I would not make it past my first birthday, later on in life I have realized that I chose to believe in something different. I have to believe that there is a purpose in my life and that I made it through this far for a reason. What I have learned is that people want to bring you down because they don't see how it is going to happen and work it out and why you want to move away from the crowd.

They don't want you to move. You have already made them feel uncomfortable by thinking differently that when they hear you want to try something new and go in a different direction, they figure out a trap to keep you in so you stay where you are.

Critics are great. Welcome them and get fired up. It means that you are doing something right. Any kind of success generated will attract attention. Even greater success will attract more problems. That is what you want to have. If you do not have bigger problems to solve, then you are not moving towards success fast enough. Most people have this backwards. They think that if they face criticism, they are doing something wrong. Look, critics are just confused admirers. If you retreat back and allow the naysayers dictate how you live, then you have let them win. The winner has to be you. Win by succeeding. Win by striving for greatness. A paradigm is much like a critic. It is your inner critic. Your mind will tell you all sorts of reasons why you should go back to living how you were used to.

I will tell you a real life example right now that I have experienced. This morning a friend of mine dragged me to a weight loss meeting for support. Clearly I do not need the program, but she does. After sitting through an hour meeting and hearing a dozen of testimonials, she asked me what she should do. I just answered her in the best way I knew how.

"Look, you are here now. Make a decision and stick to it. Take action. What will it be?"

The team leader was surprised by my response and how straight forward I was with my friend. No matter what program that you choose to pursue, make a decision. Whether it's our program at <u>Vivian Fitness</u> or something else, make a decision and stick to it.

Here is the lesson learned about paradigms. Your mind will tell you all the reasons why you shouldn't. If you figured what you want in life, move past that programming and take action. Take that initial step towards your goal and keep taking those steps until you have conditioned yourself to move past fear.

When you decide to go on the raw food diet, don't let others tell you that you have lost your mind and that eating raw foods is something bad for your health. For a moment is step away from them and observe what they are eating and how they are feeling. Ask yourself, "If they keep eating the same way that they are now, how would their life look like five years from now?" That will surely give you some perspective.

Listen, you have probably done more damage to your body by drinking coffee, eating potato chips and meat all your life. A few good servings of vegetable juice and fruits is only going to make your body thank you. Don't listen to the masses. They have always been wrong. They have always accepted being average as something great. They will never be great because they are not wired to think that way. Step up and step out of being average. You do not belong there.

"Our doubts are traitors and make us lose the good we oft might win by fearing to attempt."—William Shakespeare.

It is not the particular habit that gets in the way of our success, but how you would feel if you were to change the habit? We are all creatures of habit and one thing that we don't like is change. If you are in the habit of doubting your abilities, then you will never try. If you are in the habit of filling your mind with successful thoughts, then you are sure to win.

Whatever you think about you become and whatever you focus on you become it. **Diets do not fail. People fail themselves.**

They believe that for a brief moment that they can achieve their goal by losing weight and then the second week rolls around and they have given up. That's what happens when people don't prepare themselves mentally. You can't get something for nothing. So here is your assignment.

Write down clearly the goal that you want to achieve. Next, don't give any thought of how you are going to do it. Focus on how you can. I suggest writing out this statement and carrying it with you wherever you go:

"I am so happy and grateful now that..."

Then sign your name to it. Carry it with you wherever you go.

When I first started implementing the raw foods into my diet, I made the mistake of analyzing everything. I was reading what other people have done and how they lost weight. That only confused me and just over two weeks, I gave up. It's like going to a book store and searching for a book on how to be successful in life. Of course, many people have written on this subject, so how can you choose which technique will work for you?

The simplest way is by looking at the results generated and living vicariously through the actions of others and using your intuition. Intuition helps you move through all the clutter and filter out what works and what does not. By learning how to use your intuition and asking the right questions, you will learn and understand what your body needs and you will no longer have issues with certain cravings.

If we can just become more aware and pay attention to the signals our body is telling us, we can start moving in the right direction. However, if you have never used your intuition, it can be difficult at first. Most people shut down this intellectual faculty for two reasons. At some point in their lives they were told to think logically.

Logic and intuition are like water and fire. There are on two different sides of the spectrum. When you feed your body low vibrational foods, (cooked and processed foods) you clog up the ability to read energy and pick up energy. Clean and light foods give us peace of mind.

Chapter Three

Here is a helpful tip that I have learned from one of my mentors when it comes to goal setting and goal achieving. Not only has this technique help me advance in life, but it helped me connect to the infinite source of supply. You see, we live in an abundant world. Everything is available to us. All we have to do is learn how to ask the right questions and be quiet to hear the answer.

Ask for guidance throughout the day. Before you can put clean food in your body, a deep cleanse is in need. To have results that you want on the raw food diet, you need to do three things. The first is detoxing. The second is cleansing and the last is rebuilding.

Here is a fun fact that would get you thinking for years of what you have been eating all this time and get you on the pathway to living a healthier lifestyle.

Based on the research study done by Paul Kouchakoff, when eating fifty-one percent more cooked foods, the body will react to the food as if it's a foreign organism. Simply put, if you eat more cooked foods, the level of your white blood cells increase and your body is fighting off the food that you have just eaten. Scary right?

See, for a very long time, medical professionals have been taught to treat symptoms of a patient, but if you ask them how to cure disease. They don't have the slightest idea of how to do it. I can vouch for myself here.

When I had liver disease, the first thing that the doctors told me is to go on this dangerous chemotherapy treatment. Out of fear and not really thinking and looking for alternative ways to restore my life, I took on the treatment without looking at the side effects. I mean we have always been there, haven't we—when a doctor comes back in the room and you think of how you are going to get out of this mess. When I have come to the end of my rope and knew that the side effects were too much for me to handle, I started looking for a better way. I don't know if you are the type of person who is reading this book as the last resort and searching for answers, but all I know is that the medical approach does not work. What I am suggesting is that you explore your options and try something different. Take on a holistic approach instead of the medical approach.

(These statements are from my personal experience only. Please consult your doctor or medical professional if you have any questions about your health and wellbeing. I will not be held liable for any personal experience shared about my health and what steps I have taken to better my lifestyle choices)

This is a paradigm shift for people. Just to give you an example, I am working with a client of mine now and I am happy that I have found her because she is taking on so many medications for her problems and there are many bad side effects.

Nothing seems to work and doctors are playing guess work on her. I have been teaching her that the body already knows what is deficient in her body and what it needs. All you need to do is listen to your intuition and start introducing raw organic fruits and vegetables.

On a side note, the body cannot read labels. It only knows what it absorbs. So many people opt in for the organic label and take pill supplements, but all that organic means is that they don't use pesticides. It has nothing to do with what is in the soil and how nutrient dense it is.

You see, the whole industry of wellness and preventive health is in the business to help you feel better physically and I am a big supporter in wellness. This is why when I take a look at the scope of wellness products out there on the market today, I have to go with the top premium supplements that are the gold standard of wellness.

Click here to check out the clinical studies: http://fave.co/ 1M8EyQy

What we are here to talk about is wellness and how you can improve the quality of your life. You also have to ask yourself what has worked in the past and what improvements can be made. History does repeat itself, but we also believe that the future can be improved by learning from history.

What has worked for eighty plus years is supplementation. About fifty percent of the population knows that they need to supplement. Of course, most of them are still running on the old model of the pill delivery system, and that is where we come in. The body has a hard time recognizing pill intake, but when you introduce a high quality liquid supplement that has proven track record, that gets people's attention.

As we have mention before, **your body cannot read labels. Your body only knows what it absorbs.** A liquid delivery system is so much more powerful to be able to get your body 63 trillion cells the nutrition that it needs to be able to perform.

Nowadays, there is so much science behind liquid supplementation and behind helping families in need. You can help families avoid health challenges that they face today.

Click on the link to take the next step: http://fave.co/ 1M8EHDr

Chapter Four

The body can heal itself. The body is one of the smartest machines known to man. If the body is sick, the white blood cells rush in to make it better. If there is a cut or wound, the immune system is strong enough to restore it. The body is designed to know what it's doing to keep you alive and sustain life. However, our minds got off track of what is healthy and what is pure and as a side effect, the body stops operating like the strongest fat burning machine that it is.

Listen, we can battle this until the cows come home, but what I know for sure is that if you put nutrient dense foods in your body, the body will start working in the way that it should and eventually start repairing every cell and every tissue in your body. Just like you are the product of your environment, the environment that you create for your body is important too.

Every month, every molecule in your body is replaced. Think about what that means. Everything is replaced in your body. The skin on your hands is replaced every thirty days and the inside of your stomach every six weeks is made anew. You were a different person last month, than you are this month and the only reason you are the way that you are and the environment is the way that is it for you is because you are not willing to do anything about it to change.

The only way that we are going to fix health care in this country is not in politics and this is not a political book, so don't send me letters on this. Health starts in the kitchen and it starts with what is in front of your plate. It is time to make a shift in your beliefs of what you think is healthy and what you can do to change your health if it's not.

Since the 1930s and the rave of the fast food industry, people have been starving. An oxymoron to say since one-third of the population is obese and America has been going hungry daily.

The foods that we once had are not the same anymore and researchers now say that the parents are going to outlive their children. How scary is that? When making this convenient seemed to make things easier for the average

America is now causing each household more problems not only in their health but in their finances as well.

Did you know that on an annual basis 652,486 deaths are caused by heart disease and that 533,888 people are dying from cancer? Those numbers seem staggering and shocking because those deaths could have been avoided.

Again, this book is made not to convert you to becoming a vegetarian or going 100% raw, but it's simply to do this—to share a message of hope with the nation and to be able to provide solutions to people who have been searching for them. What we are doing here is helping you see that there are real answers out there and people that are out there every day ready to help you get underway with your own personal transformation.

It is not about how much weight you lose or what healthy habit you are going to instill in yourself, but how strong are you going to become at the end of your journey. Are you going to push yourself forward when you think you can't? It is about developing your inner strength and seeing what you are capable of doing.

Not too long ago I was sitting on the plane heading back home from a long trip and I was sitting next to these two women who were obese and I didn't say anything but I noticed what they were eating. They brought with them two massive bags of potato chips and soda and they told me it was a healthy lunch. Of course it was an overnight flight and I didn't want to get into a conversation with them, but it made me think of how brainwashed people really are. It also made me think about how food has a powerful effect on why people get food addictions in the first place.

Food addiction does not just manifest. It happens over time with certain kinds of food that alter the vibration of the body.

Sugar and caffeine are just a few examples that can potentially trigger addictions and compulsive eating.

This book is not about taking away your favorite foods, but rather give you some powerful tools that you can use daily to empower you to make new choices. The most obvious is this; you need to avoid soda and all those sugary drinks.

Although this transformation is going to be dramatic, it's not going to be done in a dramatic way. It is something that is easy and something anyone can do. Most importantly, it is affordable and convenient to your lifestyle.

People these days are so far from the truth that sometimes when an answer is right in front of them, they reject it. Frequently without realizing it people are depositing into their bodies toxins and waste that they are not even aware of how a healthy body should feel like. If you are not detoxifying the liver, you cannot process or absorb nutrients for your body.

The best way to detox is to use a method that supports the liver function while it removes impurities, but it also provides you with a clinically proven blend of vitamins and minerals as well as antioxidant phytonutrients that enhances your immunity overall.

Here is what I supplement with: http://j.mp/vhealthy
Cleansing begins with juicing. The best juicer I can recommend for you to use is the Omega 8006. Not only does it juice wheatgrass, but all of your favorite vegetables like kale, spinach, dandelions and all sorts of abundant fruit.

As a bonus, you can also make your own homemade organic nut butter. Here are a few rules of thumb: Drink at least half your body weight in ounces of water per day. Avoid as much meat and soy products as possible.

Exercise at least three times a week for about ten minutes and have alkaline foods in the morning to boost your energy throughout the day.

When we change the way we eat and begin the process of transforming our body, we can also start the process of healing ourselves on an emotional level and how the world sees us. I believe that there is a global shift happening on the planet where people are starting to wake up and become more aware of who they are. People are starting to realize that they are more than just their physical self.

This leads me to my next statement which is; when you change the energy of how you show up in the world, you will bend the Universe at will. All healing of any kind, whether it is from emotional scarring, compulsive eating or addictions, all starts on a spiritual level, not the physical. Healing starts with an intention and not from a head-space.

Chapter Five

Here is where I get spiritual on you. Some of you will either skip this chapter or continue reading. Regardless of what you do, you need a spiritual backbone to everything that you do. Have faith in something.

Mahatma Gandhi said it best—"be the change that you want to see in the world."

If you become the change that you want, other people will see that and would like to do what you do. Positive change is always good for us and for the planet. What you do today with your health can set off a positive momentum for other people and you can be the example that sets it all in.

When I embarked on this journey to find health and happiness, I kind of stumbled on raw foods and I guess that it found me. It's great when you start searching for answers and then it finds you at the perfect time just when you need it. So how did I get here? If it wasn't clearly laid out in front of me already of what my destiny would be, I needed to test it out a couple of times.

My story is this—I was born at twenty-four weeks, paralyzed from the waist down and was told that I would not make it past my first birthday. By the time I was eighteen years old, I had more than enough career changes than anyone can have in a lifetime. I was working as a nutritionist, then as a personal trainer, a professional body builder, photographer, real estate developer and among other jobs that could easily fill this book. The chaos and stress of trying to balance my life flipped upside down on the day that I found out that I had liver disease. I got here by painting myself into a corner.

I got myself here by not realizing that I needed to slow things down and pay attention to what my body was telling me. I ended up making myself sick. Stress piled up on my life and because I was trying to figure out what diet works I used myself as the test subject. I have tried over twenty different diet plans and programs and even took some diet pills. All of that stress and change of diets caused a series of problems in my body and I started to feel weak and got sick often.

Albert Schweitzer once said that we are just treating symptoms and not really the cause of the disease. We need to look at the person from a holistic point of view. This is what I have missed out on even though I was in the fitness industry. I have missed out on using my intuition to help me and direct me on what is really going on beneath the surface.

After centuries, you would think that people would get this right. People are moving faster and faster away from what is healthy and being blinded by what are more convenient for them. Now if you look at the average American, most of their lives spent at work and sleeping. Their lives do not circulate what is important to them most like their family, friends and their health.

So here I was at eighteen lying in bed thinking this was the end. I was diagnosed with liver disease. From that point, my philosophy changed and I started to look at alternative ways to heal my body and did research on what caused the disease first. The solution was simple. I needed to go on a detox diet.

Here is my new philosophy. Food is not supposed to make you feel drained, cranky and irritated. It is the complete opposite and I really didn't get that until I started detoxing my body.

Hypocrites nailed it when he said that, "Let food be your medicine and medicine be your food."

Food in the purest form like raw foods is there to rebuild the body and nurture it back to health. This is God's gift to us. Food was never meant to be grilled, stir fried, broiled or baked. Tell me, have you ever found flour or bread in nature?

Have you ever seen a chimp eat a piece of toast with eggs and bacon? No. You will not find that in nature. If you can't find it in nature in the purest form, then you should not eat it.

So simple.

If it moves and it's alive and you have to cook it, stay away. Whatever is green and it grows in nature and it reproduces itself in the soil, you want that. See, you can know all the benefits of eating raw foods and the dangers of eating fast food and you can still be the sickest person in the room. Information is not that helpful. Information gets us nowhere if it is not applied. I'm not here to give you more information that you can put away in your life. What I am here to do is make you realize that food—any type of food has an energetic quality to it.

There are enzymes in every food particle that you can consume and you need those to sustain life.

When you eat cooked foods, the digestive enzymes then have to work hard to help you digest the food. For them it's like running against the wind. Your body eventually gives out from all the resistance and the immune system breaks down from toxic build up. When that happens, you are in the danger zone. Get this, the white blood cells and the immune system sees every food that you eat, which is processed and cooked as an alien in the body. Guess what happens next?

This is fifth grade biology here. The body's defense army rushes in to attack the invader. Isn't that wild? So when you eat fifty-one percent more cooked foods, not only are you not getting valued nutrition, but you are encouraging the body to break down faster which then causes premature aging, cancer, diabetes, and high numbers in cholesterol and blood pressure.

Do you see where I am getting with this?

Food that you take on that is more acid like meat and dairy, coffee included weakens the body. By the way, eating animal protein to gain muscle mass is a complete myth. When you eat a dead animal you are taking on their cholesterol and their disease and fat.

Our bodies are not meant to digest animal protein. Why do you think you feel tired after eating a big Thanksgiving meal or having a piece of steak? Again, food provides us with energy and not drains us from it and I could go into all the details of what vitamin you need and what minerals do to the body, backed by some powerful knowledge in science, but really that is not my style and not my approach to things. I like to keep things simple.

In the discoveries that I have made when using my intuition to guide me on what kinds of food will support my body and by working with clients, I have found that there are three sabotaging pillars.

These sabotaging pillars prevent you from ever having any success in dieting or getting to your target weight goal.

Chapter Six

The first sabotaging pillar is obvious—food. From working with my clients every day and new clients that I come across my path, I have noticed that they are using food as an excuse to why They are where they are and not even realizing the amount of damage they are causing long term.

Here is what I mean. You can either have empowering beliefs of how you treat your body and what foods you feed your body or you can have disempowering beliefs and live in your story. Many people today are living in the past and not putting enough leverage on themselves to change.

If your current circumstances are causing you more pain but then you are not doing anything about them, then you haven't got a strong enough association to why you must change. If you learn how to use pain to your advantage, you can overcome any obstacle. I am not just saying that to give you hope and encouragement.

I am teaching you how to leverage your excuses so that you can develop stronger associations to why things must change and now and why you are not making decisions to do anything about that. Here's what happens to most people.

They start off on a diet and everything is going great until that mysterious circumstance happens and they reach for their comfort food to avoid the problem—too common for many Americans I believe. Instead of using food as a drug to numb the pain, identify what you are facing instead of eating your problems away. The answer is not to eat. The answer is to overcome. Ask yourself this—Am I really that hungry or am I just reaching for food instead of avoiding the things I should be facing?

What I have also seen in various weight loss meetings is that once a client loses weight, they need an excuse to justify why they deserve that dessert. It's as if they feel they are punishing themselves for eating healthy and not giving themselves what they want. They want instant gratification. They want a reason to fall of their success path to losing weight. Why this happens, I will never understand. Even at these weight loss meetings I ask the client why they feel they need a whole bag of chips or ten gallons of ice cream.

(I am not making this up. I heard this yesterday when my friend brought me to one of those meetings)

One individual claimed that she needed it. It was something she was going to do for herself. She felt like she deserved it, but then felt guilty for gaining five pounds that week.

As this chapter comes to a close, let me tell you a secret about success. You will never have it if you are not willing to pay the price for the promise. The price could be many things. It could be ignoring that fridge full of ice cream at the store and opting in for some salad instead. It is sacrificing ten minutes of your time to exercise no matter how busy your schedule looks like. It is about making that commitment to yourself and sticking to it. When you say to yourself that you want to lose fifteen pounds, do it. Don't wait and don't delay. Delay directs denial.

Do it now. I mean right now. Close this book and take action. Put that ice cream down or that cup of coffee. Here is where I will probably receive even more criticism for this book. I will probably hear that I have not given you a step by step guide to how to lose weight and feel awesome.

You do not need a step by step guide. All you need is someone behind you to scream RUNNNNNNN!!!! Take action. Any kind of action that will move you forward.

The intent of this book was to help you understand why raw foods is a good option and how food addictions start. It was about providing you the information you need to understand how your brain works and how you are always in control of what you do. There are three pillars of sabotage because there are three things that happen when you get off target. Food choices will always be number one.

The second sabotaging pillar is emotions. Your emotions have a heavy influence just as much as the environment on your psyche. If you want to transform your life and your want to transform your body, you have to work from within and work on yourself.

Change you first and change your thinking. Food is energy and your thoughts are energy. Since they are the same, whatever thought you have, you will attract to you the vibrational food that corresponds to that thought. Why do you think you reach for greasy food instead of the salad when you are stressed?

When you are not feeling your best, you will find yourself out of control. You will allow any emotion to rule your life. Remember that you are the master of your own fate. You at any given moment can control what you do and how you feel. Therefore, learn how to master your feelings.

Someone with prior experience with food addiction or compulsive eating will understand this to be true. When you are in a positive frame of mind, you make good choices. When you are not, you are not. The key is to gain awareness. Understand what you are doing and why.

The third pillar is the environment. Sure, you can have the will power with food and the emotions, but the only reason why raw foods are not going to work for you is if you sneak in plate fills of cooked foods and have a guilt day. Listen, I am not against spoiling yourself rarely, but cheating yourself out of perfect health is another deal. Not long ago I was in Vegas on a business trip and I have met a well-known doctor that if I mentioned his name you would know who he is. What stood out from the whole conversation is what he had said.

"The environment pulls the trigger….that causes you to be overweight."

Everywhere that you go you see fast food places and meals that have too much sodium in it, GMO, high fructose corn syrup, and chemicals that you can't even pronounce. Your environment shapes you and you shape into the environment and unless you do something about it and mold the environment the way that you want it, healthcare is not going to be the same. The power to true health and wellness is in the decisions that you make and what you choose. Decide to transform your body and transform your life and I will be there with you through the hard times and your victories celebrating with you.

I thank you for allowing me to be your transformation life coach. Finally, we would love to see you in our future events and retreats and we hope that our paths cross one day. Until next time, live with purpose every day of your life and expect abundance in your life.

The next following chapters that you are going to read are the second publication of No More Diets.

Chapter Seven

This publication will hold a real glimpse into the raw food diet and how effective it is on a long term basis. Also, as mentioned in the introduction, the following chapters will reveal the top three flaws that were found in the system and why.

As of today, our clients still embrace the system of being on the raw food diet and understanding the difference between acid and alkaline, however in reality are not vegetarians or 100% raw foodies. In this section I will explain why that it is so and give you a more realistic approach towards healthy living.

Be sure to visit us on our website via www.VivianFitness.com

Here is the truth. Being on a raw good diet is time consuming.

Realistically speaking, going to the raw food diet for a short time to jolt and shock the body to go into a cleanse to get rid of impurities and move towards going into a more alkaline state is useful. Recommendations for going on the raw food diet for a short time would be beneficial and I would suggest reading further into the book to discover what acid and alkaline does to the body if you are not in harmony.

As for being time consuming and darn right expensive if you are the type of person that is always on the go, raw foods and juicing is not going to work out in the long run. At first it was nice juicing some fresh organic carrots in the morning and the weekends when your days is not as rushed as the others, but when work rolls around the corner, the last thing that you want to do is pull out that juicer and squeeze some kale leaves into the mix and wait for it to go through it's process. In a few raw books, it is recommended to freeze your juices until you are ready to use them, but who has time for that?

Now this chapter is not about being lazy and making excuses. It is about being real and giving you a real insight to weight loss and why most people fail even on the first day. As I said before, diets do not fail on people. People fail themselves. That is absolutely true, but I am also here to be authentic with you and give you my insight of why I am no longer doing any kind of liquid diet, raw food diet or even considering going on "a diet" ever again.

Just thinking about how I have to restrict the kinds of food I eat and when I eat them and then having another to-do-list is impractical. When you are out and about you are not going to run back home so you can juice your organic greens, nor are you going to program your life around your new found diet. Honestly, that is what I did when I have gone on this raw food craze.

I've also juiced during the hot dog days of summer so freshness was my number one concern. Yes, going raw would save you money on your grocery bill, but that is if you stay home all day and not go out. As you can tell, already it seems like a pain to be on a raw food diet and this is why I no longer recommend people to go on a raw food diet unless you can fit it into your schedule.

Making that commitment is tough and you won't go there. On average person won't go there just for the thrills. Here is another reason why raw foods are time consuming or at least from my perspective, it was consumed for the long term. It's just not realistic to or even sane to go on a full liquid diet for the rest of your life.

As in the revision of this section of the No More Diets book I received a message from a friend who was on a weight loss program. I say, "Was" because she has just sent me this message on Facebook:

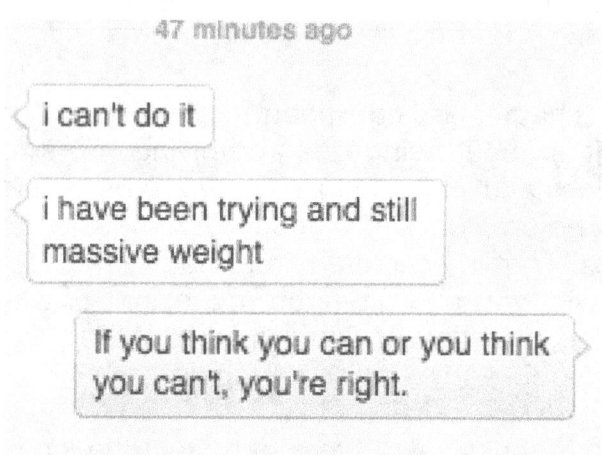

47 minutes ago

i can't do it

i have been trying and still massive weight

If you think you can or you think you can't, you're right.

I could have responded with something like, "Why do you think that is" or "tell me more about that." I have decided to go with the good ol' Henry Ford quote and leave it at that.

She was not one of my clients, just a friend who wanted to know what I was doing to keep in shape and stay in shape. Listen, a healthy lifestyle is not for everybody. You really have to put in the work and make it work. It doesn't matter what program you are on or what "diet" you are following, if you will not persist, you will not win. End of story.

From the perspective of a person who has been there as well, I can tell you that the journey is not easy. It is tough. It is hard. Most of the time you just want to give up and not press forward. However, the journey is worth it!

It will be worth all the struggles that you have to go through to become better and stronger. When I was stuck on a goal and wanted to quit at some point, my mentor would tell me,

"Boss up and take ownership. The bigger the struggle, the bigger the success."

Successful people move past fear. They move past pain and go through the unimaginable to come up on top. Why do I tell you this?

First off, I am fired up more than ever when I get these responses on my Facebook page. It just tells me the kind of commitment that person made to themselves about fitness and living a healthier lifestyle. It gets me fired up even more to know that they already gave up in their mind.

If you are going after what you want, quitting is never an option. It never enters your mind. You will persist until you get what you want. You have to develop a lion mentality. Be relentless. Be furious. Be determined and ignore the opinions of others. You have to be willing to go alone. Many who started with you won't finish with you.

Right now, I am prepping for the WBFF fitness competition. Let me tell you, the work I have to put in is unreasonable. The mental struggle is hard but I keep on pushing forward. Every day that I accomplish a new goal, is another victorious day. There will be days where I feel I am not progressing, but I know I will hit my target eventually.

Follow me here on Bodybuilding.com to see my progress.
http://bodyspace.bodybuilding.com/vivianfitness

Also, I will be posting progress reports monthly on my blog:
http://VivianFitness.com/about

Chapter Eight

Another flaw about the raw food diet and any diet is that it's confined.

Can you imagine how much is out there today that can be classified in the "acid" food group as opposed to being in the alkaline? Just looking at the chart would overwhelm you and if you have compulsive behaviors, what you would do is be very straight-laced with the process. Your meal has to be exactly 90% raw foods and hydrate at least half your body weight in ounces. Being so in control with your diet will first of all make you crazy and second of all get you in the behavior of developing eating disorders, even if it is eating healthy. Measuring everything exactly is not the way to live. Not everything has to be exact and to the point in your eating. Having a meal should be enjoyed and not stressed over.

When I have leaned off of going raw and got out of my trance, I have noticed that the raw food "gurus" and health nuts out there pushed the idea of incorporating "super foods" and they made it seem that if you do not include them in your smoothie, it's the end of the world. Pathetic.

Now my philosophy is this: have a drink of greens in the morning and minimize the amount of acid foods that you have. Keep your food groups balanced throughout the day and you should be okay.

If you do your research, many raw food coaches were somewhat vocal about not being able to eat meat and protein and claimed that we receive our protein from the veggies that we eat. And do not get me started with the frequent colonics and water fasting.

Raw food restaurants seem to be healthy but what I have found through my research is that most of their food is bland, dehydrated and made into nut spreads. Raw food restaurants were beginning to Americanize and blend in with the culture. That simply does not work. Having a colorful salad with protein is healthy, but having foods that are dried up and have no nutrients in them is not healthy at all. You might as well go to a fast food place instead.

However one thing that is great about raw foods is that it teaches you how to combine your foods the right way. Here is what I mean. Throughout my book I have mentioned to you that it's not that most people are over fat, but most people are over acid.

Here are the basic rules to follow when having a meal and how this combination can potentially help you boost your metabolism, burn fat and give you the ultimate energy throughout the day. I have learned this method from Kimberly Snyder, The Beauty Detox Solution.

Do Not Combine In The Same Meal:
- *Protein And Fruit*
Fruit takes on average fifteen to thirty minutes to digest as opposed to protein which can take up to four hours.

- *Protein And Starch*
Protein and starch combined in one meal like meat and potatoes can also slow down digestion and cause bloating. If you are going to have protein and starch in the same meal, have a salad first and then the starch followed by the protein.

Starches need an alkaline base the digest (this is why having the salad first to coat the stomach breaks down the

41

starch faster) and the protein needs an acid base to break down. Since protein and starches are at opposite charge, they cancel each other out, causing lack of digestion.
- *Protein And Protein*
This can cause toxic build up in your body and slow down the process of your digestion.

Combine In The Same Meal:
- Protein And Vegetables

Another Option To Creating a Healthy Meal Plan:
Carb-Cycling first originated and used for bodybuilders and in the practical world, it was too mainstream to understand. Now, carb-cycling is made easy. Eat small meals throughout the day, preferably every two hours and alternate what you eat throughout the week.

To better understand the carb-cycling solution so you can apply it to your life today, I highly recommend reading and implementing Chris Powell's incredible book Choose More To Lose More For Life.

Here is the best part of the carb-cycling solution, you get to eat a lot! No more counting calories. No more breaking commitments to yourself about starting the diet on Monday when what you really are saying is that you are not sure if you ever want to start. No more time consuming recipes that do not work at the end. Choose More To Lose More is all about giving you a realistic solution to looking and feeling great without ever being on a diet!

We all need support now and again. So here is your chance to receive it. We have spoke about the principle of never being on a diet and never going on a fad diet, because we all know how well those turn out. Millions of people around the world struggle with their weight and are looking for answers that will not only give them success in the short run, but long term results that they can enjoy for a lifetime.

With the Carb-Cycling Solution, you are in control and you have the tools right at your finger tips! Take a look at the illustration below as the tools guide you and direct you to exactly what you need to do to feel better and be healthier.

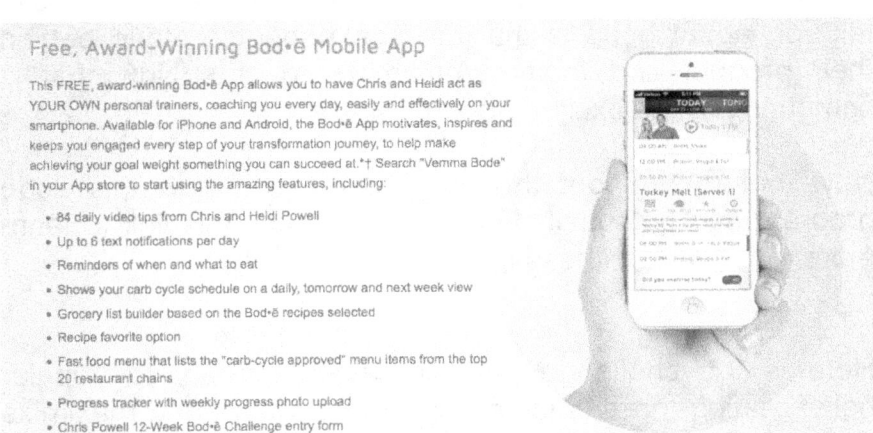

Free, Award-Winning Bod•ē Mobile App

This FREE, award-winning Bod•ē App allows you to have Chris and Heidi act as YOUR OWN personal trainers, coaching you every day, easily and effectively on your smartphone. Available for iPhone and Android, the Bod•ē App motivates, inspires and keeps you engaged every step of your transformation journey, to help make achieving your goal weight something you can succeed at.*† Search "Vemma Bode" in your App store to start using the amazing features, including:

- 84 daily video tips from Chris and Heidi Powell
- Up to 6 text notifications per day
- Reminders of when and what to eat
- Shows your carb cycle schedule on a daily, tomorrow and next week view
- Grocery list builder based on the Bod•ē recipes selected
- Recipe favorite option
- Fast food menu that lists the "carb-cycle approved" menu items from the top 20 restaurant chains
- Progress tracker with weekly progress photo upload
- Chris Powell 12-Week Bod•ē Challenge entry form

So many people ask me what am I doing today that is relevant, simple and easy to use. This is it. The Bode award-winning app is my secret weapon to dropping those 30 pounds in 30 days and keeping it off! You see, losing weight anyone can do, but how many can sustain those results? Studies have shown that people who go on a diet either gain the weight back, plus two more pounds or fail succeed.

This revolutionary approach to wellness is a story that has never been told before. This 12-week challenge is about being different while still being yourself. What we mean by that is, you are still going to enjoy the foods that you love, just on different days.

You are never going to feel deprived or feel like you are sacrificing things that you love. That is what No More Diets is essentially about too. With Bode, you will learn about this proven method of carb-cycling and how it can help you boost your metabolism and burn fat without ever feeling like you are dieting. This is your best chance to reach your weight loss goal. I can tell you from experience that this is a program that I fully endorse and happily promote because it works! I have seen so many programs and products out there in the fitness industry that it can make your head spin. Most of them are just hype and clever marketing. What I can tell you about bode is that the spokespeople stand behind their product and their commitment to you. Now that is something to get excited about!

Now, before you get this, let me tell you how this bode program can potentially work for you. Click this link to learn more: http://vivianfitness.com/24plan/

Here is the challenge that we face. Contrary to popular belief, eating three times a day to lost weight and maximize your fat burning potential is not enough. Most people eat large heavy meals throughout the day, which causes the metabolism to slow down. That means that by eating inconsistently throughout the day accelerates the natural production of cortisol. Cortisol is known for triggering the desire to binge eating and storing belly fat!

This program helps you build the necessary habits where you get to eat smaller meals more often. Not only will this help you fight those hunger pains, but fuel your body to let go of the necessary belly fat you have been storing.

As a bonus, The Get Fit Coaching Program along with the Bode Plan teaches you how to alternate carbs throughout the week to keep your metabolism running. Instead of the typical eat less meals and replace it with a shake or a bar, you get to eat more often and the foods that you love.

Did you know that the body responds well when different variety of foods are introduced? That also means that the body responds positively to carbs when combined with a balanced assortment of healthy fruits, vegetables, protein and fats. Let's also remind you that the program incorporates a cheat-day once a week. How cool is that?

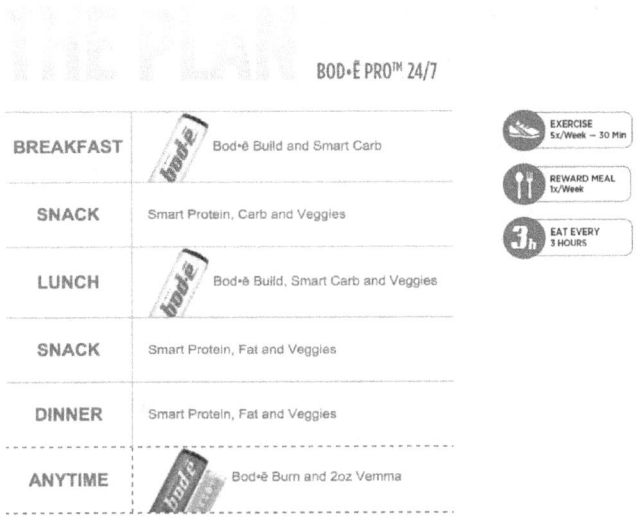

That is how the plan looks like. Of course it can be customized to your liking and FREE meal plans and recipes with guided instruction of the portion size.

It has never been easier and convenient to have this available to you.

When I first was introduced to the Bode Plan, I got excited. I knew that this was something that can work for me. I've tried different kinds of diets and fad diets. Nothing really worked as great as Bode did.

Honestly, I see myself incorporating this plan in my everyday life because it's simple. The meals are planned out for you and the app texts you on your phone when it is time to eat.

There are constant positive reminders of how well you are doing. Plus with the ability to track my progress right on my smartphone is amazing. With some tweeks to the Bode Plan, I even use it today to prepare for my fitness competition.

To take the next step and be apart of this Get Fit Coaching Program, visit my website: http://vivianfitness.com/coaching contact me directly on Facebook. I will help you get started in the same way that I have.

Chapter Nine

What happens between the point where someone goes through a transformation, maintains it for a short time and then goes back to their habitual routine and calls it quits? We all had our moments of victories where we feel great about our bodies, and then there are those moments where you stare in the mirror one day and wonder what the heck happened?

Everyone that I know or even read about always talks about their successes, but I am more curious about failure when it comes to dieting. Here are the top five challenges, according to my friend Dmitry who considered going on a diet and for a short while trying out the raw food diet. It would be easier to just give you a philosophical approach to how diets, including the raw food diet is contradicting but it's more useful and helpful to you hearing it from first hand experience.

Getting Started:
"It's not the question of doing the right thing or the wrong thing. People are afraid of the unknown and they stick with a product or service that they are comfortable with."

Consistency:
In my interview with Dmitry, I have challenged him to think about why do people do what they do and why they fail to take action. You see, we are creatures of habit and we like completion.

Even though something may be good for us and good for other people, doesn't mean that we are going to get up and do the thing that we say we are going to do. If there is not enough leverage on the person to make the change that they say they want, they are going to fall into their old patterns. It's silly to go into your garden and say, "There are no weeds."

Thinking that way will sabotage the garden. People are always consistent with their identity of who they think they are.

Overcome Addiction:
"When you psychologically prepare yourself, then that will lead you to other steps. Life in general is a struggle between overcoming obstacles and the things that we are used to. At first it was a lie that I am not out of the addiction, but I am proud of myself that I stopped. First, you have to be truthful that you have an addiction and make a positive choice and a decision."

Fooling Yourself:
"It's not about the win. It's the involvement. You have to trick yourself into believing that you can do it. Incorporate every action to thinking positive.

Honesty:
I wouldn't be human if I didn't have any flaws and struggles just like everyone else. In the interview I have mentioned that even though I make the effort to eating healthy everyday, the one thing that I am falling back on is doing my "Hour of Power." It is a ritual I used to do every morning before starting my day and it consisted of going for a walk or a jog for an hour while listening to Tony Robbins. I love what Dmitry mentioned at the end.

"Are you really happy with yourself?"

If you would take away all of these challenges to progressing in life and mastering the health aspect of your life, this one would be the top qualifier. There are so many people out there today who is just going through life just to get along and not really living. Their lives are composed of mundane rituals that drain their energy and liveliness.

So here is my challenge to you. What are the top challenges have you have in weight loss and what are the top three things you done in the past that didn't produce lasting change?

Chapter Ten

The Psychology, Physiology and Philosophy
Of Nutrition:

It is time to understand that what the billion dollar wellness industry doesn't want you to know may be the exact thing that is potentially killing you. They don't want you to know that the foods that you are eating are causing more damage than good, and it is masked by the happy marketing strategy that has got you brainwashed.

See, food has a great impact on your emotions and food is probably one of the things that is used in most cultures as a connector. Today, people are not used to having a normal conversation with a person so they use food as a communicator and a distracting at the same time when things get a little uncomfortable. Food is also used as an ice-breaker, and a conflict inhibitor, which ultimately leads to all kinds of food addictions.

One of the main food addictions comes from eating an excessive amounts of processed foods, cooked foods that are also coated with high fructose corn syrup and complex sugars. When combined, this makes a deadly pair because our bodies are not meant to digest these chemicals and fillers so we end up feeling dumbed out and drugged out.

Recent study from France (heard this on the Katie Couric Show From Dr. Hyman) revealed that sugar virtually can be eight times more addictive than cocaine. To put this in perspective which you will understand, when a person consumes large amounts of sugar and foods that contain sugar, a chemical is released into the brain that acts as a motivator. At the time sugar is being processed in the body, dopamine is being fired off excessive amounts and the brain lights up as a ping Pong machine. Every time that a person eats sugar, their brain gets happy. Soon enough the tolerance of sugar increases and it takes higher amounts, or doses of sugar-content foods to give that same reward.

We as human being is stimulated by what drives us. Those two drives are the reward of pleasure or the regret of pain. Since we want to avoid pain and gain pleasure, we are in constant search of what can we find that will give us more of those happy feelings. Moreover, after that sugar rush, stress hormones are triggered releasing adrenaline and cortisol. All in all, increasing sugar intake can also change a person's taste buds.

With enough repetition, and enough emotional references, pleasure are linked to eating foods that cause more harm than good. For example, why do people reach for food when they are in a high emotional state? It's because they have linked themselves neurologically to experience the positive emotions and hide the ones that trigger them to have emotional baggage. In such cases, food is no longer seen as medicine, but a poison to the body.

Everything now is redesigned to fit the "bigger the better" model of today's fast paced economy and with the speed that we are moving to mass production, our species will move towards mass self-destruction. These are just some psychological ideas of nutrition.

Now that we have built a foundation as to how compulsive eating and food addictions begin to form, let's move on to exploring the idea of how most people view nutrition and why the majority of people just look "fat." It's not that people are overeating per-se. It's just that they are over acid. The amount of energy you experience on a day to day basis has nothing to do with how much you eat, but rather what you eat.

We all heard of this expression, that you are what you eat and it's absolutely true. If you eat slush all day long, soon enough you will look and feel like it. There are many distinctions between over eating, under eating and simply not knowing what to do anymore nutrition wise.

As soon as someone gains a bit of weight or they are already overweight, the first thing that comes to mind is to go on a diet. Contrary to popular belief, going on a "diet" is the worst thing that you can do.

What are the first three letters in the word diet? Now you see why the majority of the population wants to avoid it. First they are motivated you see. They get on the first diet. Usually it consists of not eating anything for breakfast and just having their morning coffee, followed by a "healthy" veggie sandwich for lunch and take out for dinner. When that doesn't work on day two, here comes diet number two. This diet consists of eating heavier meals less often which causes the metabolism to slow down. Even though they are eating healthier, but in large quantities throughout the day, the body still goes into starvation mode.

This activates the natural production of cortisol, triggering the body to store belly-fat and simultaneously increasing the chances of binge eating, hunger pains and emotional eating. We have mentioned this in the previous chapter when we introduced you to the Get Fit Coaching Program.

Habitual patterns like this causes our body to get out of balance and break down. To understand this process of biological breakdown happens in our body, we need to understand what our body is and how it works. Our bodies are running on electrical currents tied with magnetism. All the nerves of your body send signals throughout your body through electricity.

Every single cell that is healthy and alive is run through these currents and it's only going to happen with a delicate balance in our biochemistry. So what does that all mean and how does this relate to you?

Well, anything that would disrupt this electrical current would slow down the process of keeping you totally energetic and alive. The more natural energy you have, (that is not chemically altered or infused by drinking caffeine) the healthier you are going to be and the younger you are going to feel.

Going green, as mentioned in the first publication of this book is the way to start the process of cleansing the body of its toxins and recharging the batteries. Acid takes us out of balance and the **number one cause of acid is human emotions.**

If you experience anger, resentment, frustration and stress on a daily basis, I can guarantee you that your body is completely out of balance.

Just as you stimulate the body to produce acid through human emotions, you can also stimulate the body to produce a more harmonious state. Here is something you need to remember. As important that the temperature of the body needs to be at 98.6, on a scale from one to fourteen, to maintain an alkaline state your blood should be slightly alkaline and at 7.36. For reference, one is pure acid.

That would burn a hole through steel and fourteen is totally alkaline. The middle range is where you want to be and close to 7.36 as possible. If you are off by a point or two, instant source of life would stop. It is like unplugging an electrical source. This is not where you want to be. The blood is also the river of life. It carries all the oxygen and nutrients in and carries all the toxins out in one sweeping motion. The red blood cells have two charges. On the outside is a negative charge and on the inside is positive. Now think for a second. When you introduce more acid to the body, first it has to figure out what to do with it and then it adds on more negative charge to the red cells. This slows them down, clump them together and making it difficult to pass through various capillaries.

Acid strips away the electrical charge of these cells, which explains why most people feel like a slush after having a heavy meal filled with mostly acid causing foods. Interestingly, when acid is introduced to the body, red blood cells begin to weaken and then eventually die off, they begin to release their own acids into the bloodstream.

This compounding effect pollutes the body, even faster causing negative momentum. On the other hand, you can be completely "healthy" but obsessive about what you are going to eat and when that just by your human emotions, you are producing acid in the internal environment.

Hence why most people do not lose weight and then try another diet to see if it works for them. Dieting is not the problem and once you understand that, you will never have to diet because you will create a positive environment internally. Diets do not work essentially. They are just a quick fix for something that is internal.

Typically it's habitual behavior. All that diets do for a short period of time is help you manage your weight until you get to a desired goal and most likely 80% of the people who have ever been on a weight loss program gained the weight back plus a few more pounds within two years. Here is why-- people like to eat.

I call this Rapid Growth vs. Gradual Improvement Effect.

Integrity and intentions are diminished when we try to cut everything out of our diet just so we and feel like we are on the right track.

The problem with this is that the we are not used to going cold turkey. Rapid growth can be compared to pushing up a heavy bolder up the mountain. It can be done, but it's hard work. Gradual improvement on the other hand is easier and takes less effort.

It's throwing all the rules out the window about what you know about dieting and nutrition and building a new model. In the next chapter you will learn a how to apply a proven system that will enable you to lose weight, burn fat, boost your metabolism and build powerful momentum behind having consistent results.

Chapter Eleven

How To Have Unstoppable Energy and
Save Big On Your Grocery Bill Of $100 a Week:

Unstoppable energy starts with not what you decide to do at the gym, but what you do in the kitchen. We all heard the expression that abs start in the kitchen and not at the gym. That is absolutely true. What you put in your body has a direct effect of how you think and what you do with your life.

Having energy also doesn't mean that you have to cut out your favorite foods either. What unstoppable energy means really is how you feel about yourself. Human emotion is the first thing that is going to determine your energy level, not your diet or how much weight you can lift and how much cardio that you do.

Human emotion and the state that you go to every single day will determine how you would feel and the kinds of decisions that you make. Moment to moment you are deciding whether this action will align you with where you want to go and the state that you are in will determine if you take action or lack of. So how do you get to the point where you are feeling vibrant, alive and totally fulfilled and fueled with passion?

Move! Emotion is created by motion. If you want to feel a certain way, put your physiology in the state where you give a command and follow through. The way that you are ever going to grow is if you expand by demand. Give yourself a target that you must follow through on and raise your standards. That is how you are going to transform your life. It's by raising our standards that we learn how to become bigger than ourselves and expect more from ourselves than anyone can ever demand from us. It is by raising our standards that we discover what we are really capable of accomplishing. We can accomplish anything, but what we are willing to do is a different story. If what we are willing to do and what we need to do is not aligned with what must happen to change our lives, transformation is inborn. This doesn't just relate to food addictions or compulsive eating. Raising our standards relates to every area of our lives.

I call it the **Six Core Influences Of Fulfillment**. These are the six core categories if you will, that we strive for completion.

Briefly, they are the mind, health, relationship, career, finances, spirituality. If any of these are unfulfilled, we feel that our life is incomplete. That doesn't mean that everything needs to be perfect. That just means that at least have your life move towards your goals and be in alignment with them.

Once we have decided to raise our standards, the next step is to decide what we are not willing to accept any more. What kind of behaviors are you not going to put up with anymore and what are you going to do to change that?

What must happen in this area of your life? What action steps are you going to take right now to move towards what you want. Saying that you "diet" starts Monday when it's mid-week is just a weak prayer and it doesn't even have faith to launch it. Saying that this goal of yours starts somewhere in the future is like shooting in the dark, hoping to hit the target. You are going to lose. Integrity is the key.

Without integrity with ourselves and keeping our promises, it doesn't matter what happens after. Breaking a promise to ourselves is the worst thing that you can do because your dignity is on the line. It's not even about the amount of weight you lose or how you are going to maintain the weight or even about the energy that you are going to receive from cleansing your body. It is about believing in yourself and committing to yourself. Often times we make commitments to others, but we rarely make them for our own selves and keep them.

Recently I've attended a conference in Toronto, Canada and the speech that Ryan Sawlsville from Extreme Makeover Weight Loss Edition moved me. He spoke about having that accountability and support system around yourself and not giving up. It's about having that magic fairy dust called belief and knowing that you are going to accomplish what you set to do.

Ryan said that for him it was not about losing the two hundred and seventeen pounds. Sure it was a nice added bonus, but it was more about the commitment that he had for himself.

What an amazing guy.

Although this is not particularly "diet" related, it sure will be in your wallet. Earlier this week I was having an interesting conversation with a financier about money management and somehow our discussion lead to how much our monthly food expense was.

I was shocked to say the least that he spends at minimum $5,000 on groceries for a family of two. This does not include the budget for in-house groceries, as to his family mostly goes out to eat every night.

Sheepishly I said that my budget and spending costs for groceries averages out to about $100-150 a week if I do not want to dine out. Yes, I buy fresh ingredients and my budget can feed up to five people with my three course gourmet meal. This conversation got me thinking. Why do so many American's spend so much money on food?

The puzzling fascination is that the people who are obese or overweight actually do not spend quite as much money on food. Frankly, they are not eating enough or they are eating the right foods at the wrong time. This is not a judgement, but a slight observation from many mornings sitting at Starbucks and cafe shops people-watching and observing what the average consumer buys. Want to know the answer to why people blindly spend money left and right on things they don't even need? Here it is. It is not about you. It's about feeding your ego.

What fuels our emotions on a day to day basis is the reputation of the ego. What is yours, hers, his, mine, and I. Everyone has grown accustomed to identifying themselves with objects that have little to no value and giving meaning to something that has no meaning at all.

When I was battling with my weight many times in my life, I've given a lot of things in my life significant meaning, like I was THAT thing. I was my home, my car, the grades I got in school, my reputation and the money in my account, and not once did I bother asking the question, "who am I really?" How many times a day do you spend defending your ego, feeding it fuel and making it stronger?

How many times a day do you spend arguing with people and wanting to win because you just have to and how many times a day do you spend thinking about how you can forgive and let go of people in your life?

Every single one of us has a different way of feeding the ego, some may be material possessions and others could be food. The real question is, who are you trying to satisfy? Who are you trying to satisfy when you have that donut or that delicious New York cheesecake or the fifth slice of the hour? Surely its not your body because your body does not want that.

So what is the point of this philosophical thinking about food and feeding the ego? My observations came to the conclusion that consumers today in the United States are not just buying things that they need, but they are over spending to fill up their lives with things they think will give them fulfillment. It is as if they are buying food to consume so that they can hide what is really going on beneath the surface.

Tips On Shopping Smart To Fattening Your Wallet:

1. Plan Out Your Weekly Meals:
We have all heard this from many people that you should never go grocery shopping when you are hungry and always keep a list. Even though this is true, who has time to write down everything that they need?

The best suggestion that I can give you is plan out your meals. Here is what I mean. Let's say that you are in the meat section of the supermarket and you plan buying chicken and beef.

Find other dishes that you can make that can complement the meat and yet be used as a separate meal on it's own. Think of this as mix and matching your wardrobe and adding accessories. You still have a great outfit and it didn't cost you as much money because you recreated a whole different look with just a few pieces.

2. Shop At The Perimeter Of The Store:
This is the best way to shop if you are in a rush and want to get things done. Imagine that the supermarket is a big box. You have the entrance and exit door on one side of the cube and then fresh ingredients on the rest of the outside walls.

Do you think it would be faster to walk around the outside walls and get what you need rather than get sunk into the maze of what is going on on the inside walls of the store?

3. Adjust and Adapt:

Here you are, in the kitchen about to make that favorite meal for your family and you just missed an ingredient. Do you drive back to the supermarket and get it or adjust and adapt?

Bingo. Use what you've got. Another thing about adjusting and adapting, not a lot of people are being conscious spenders and know where their money is going.

They are spending more money on luxuries than necessities and then wonder why they do not have enough money to pay their bills. What is more important to you? Annihilating your debt or living in poverty?

4. Ego vs your bank account:
Next time that you are in the grocery store, be mindful of what you are subconsciously grabbing for dinner. Are you grabbing those frozen dinners, even the vegetable ones, and the cut up prepackaged foods instead of fresh produce?

Think about it, a pound of beef to make meat loaf is about a couple of bucks and then a few cents for some spices. Making your own meat loaf is so much healthier since you know what is going in there and you can feed more people. What is the cost of the prepackaged deal? Approximately four dollars for a small meal that can't even feed one person.

Losing weight is not much as to what is more convenient for you as to what will nourish you. In the beginning you may not want to pack your lunches to work or make your own food the night before, but those decisions are the difference between a person of discipline and a person who is foolish. Get in the routine of making food at home and shopping smart. Not only will you feel so much better because of the food that you are feeding your body, but you will save hundreds of dollars.

FREE 7-DAY TRAINING SERIES FOR FEMALE PROFESSIONALS

Sign up for my FREE 7-day training event and learn what action steps you need to take right now to turn your weight loss goals into real results. This is your year to lose weight without dieting and it's time to say goodbye to the excuse, "The diet starts on Monday."

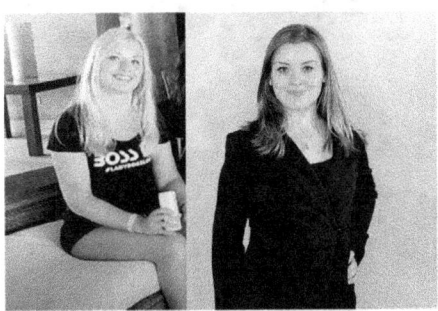 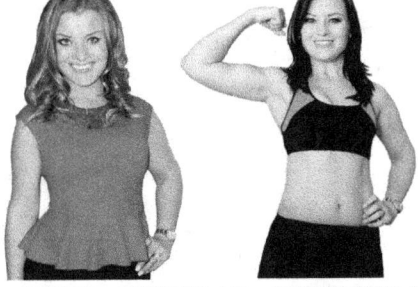

BEFORE: WEIGHT: 140   DRESS SIZE: 16   AFTER: WEIGHT: 110   DRESS SIZE: 2

Register Now *For This* FREE *Training Series* To Learn
The 7 Secrets To Never Going On A Diet Again

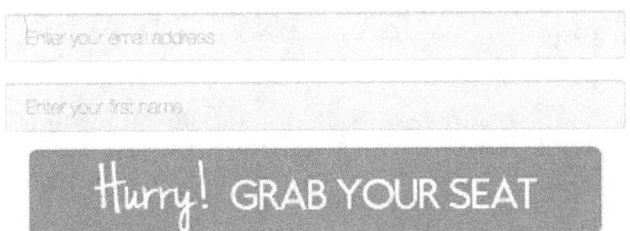

We value your privacy and would never spam you

Click <u>here</u> to register for this FREE Training Series or visit my website:

www.VivianFitness.com

GET FIT COACHING PROGRAM

MEET YOUR FITNESS TRAINER:

- Over 12+ years experience as a master life coach
- Over 10+ years experience as the top fitness trainer
- Mentored by the highest paid trainers in personal growth
- Certified Neurolinguistic Practitioner
- Certified Sports Nutrition Consultant
- Certified Reiki Master

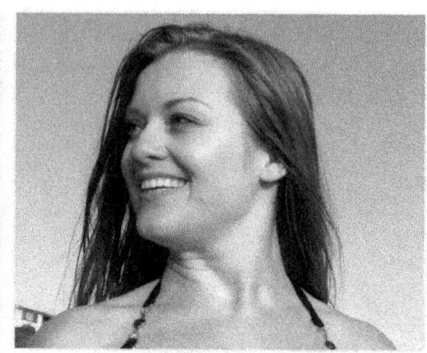

WHY I'VE DESIGNED THIS PROGRAM FOR YOU

Are you a super busy female professional who is tired of being sick and tired of getting the same results in fitness and weight loss? Have you been on a million diets too and wondered why it worked for others, but not you? Feeling confused right about now?

I've been in your shoes too many times to count, so I know how you feel. Even though I have been in the fitness industry for over 10 years, I've secretly struggled with an eating disorder and believed that if you look good on the outside then you must be "healthy."

I know that you have felt the same way. You have also tried those fad diets and felt like it was never the right fit for you for some reason. Deep down you knew going on a "diet" was unhealthy, but you did it anyway.

Here's the thing. In order for you to have an amazing life where dieting is no longer the option, you have to work on yourself. Working on you is the starting point. That is the driving force to why you do what you do. Listen, research is not going to provide you with the results you truly seek that will last. If the *real solution* was doing research and following a "diet plan," then you wouldn't feel stuck, frustrated and confused.

It's really that simple. If you want to lose weight, feel confident about yourself or even challenge yourself to see what you're capable of doing, the mindset work is super important. Without it, you'll just wonder without a real game plan set in place. You can either let your excuses stop you from getting the dream body you have always wanted or figure out why your results are the same.

FOCUS OF THE GET FIT COACHING PROGRAM

The Get Fit Coaching Program focuses on helping you develop healthy habits so that you know exactly what you need to do in order to reach your fitness goals. This program only works when you combine the proven plan with the mindset work.

You may be asking yourself, "then why do diets fail?" They don't. People fail themselves because they lack the proper support and guidance. In order for you to succeed in any endeavor, you need to have a mentor in your life that has been where you have been and gotten the results you truly desire. What I have found is that it's really the combination of investing in a high level coach, having the proven tools set in place and developing the success habits. That is the key to achieving long lasting results. Weight-loss is honestly a mind-game. Once you understand the game and how to play by the "rules," you can win.

We can all agree that we are creatures of habit. If left to our own devices without a proven direction, we drift off. That is why it is suggested for you to seek out the support you need from a high level coach to help you reach your goals.

HOW GET FIT 24/7 WORKS & WHY IT'S DIFFERENT

Click on the audio below to listen to how to get started with the Get Fit Coaching Program. Want to listen to it on your iPod, iPhone or Android? To download, right click and choose "save as."

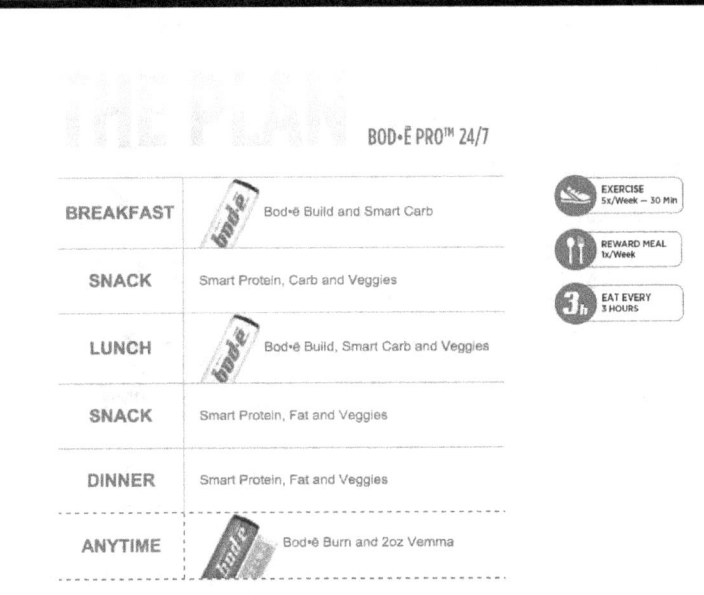

65

WHO THIS PROGRAM IS FOR

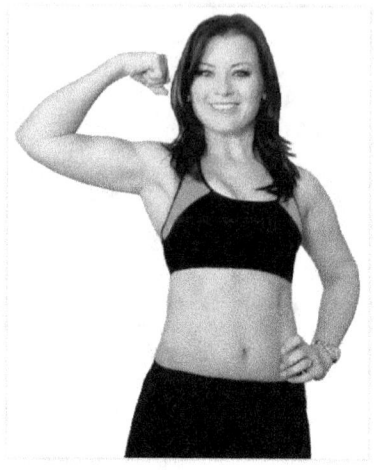

- *If you are a young female professional.*

- *If you are a (super busy) woman who is tired of being sick and tired of getting the same results.*

- *If you are the type of woman who has a strong desire for change.*

- *If you are coachable and willing to learn from a coach who has been where you are.*

- *Resolve to make time for YOU and workout at least 5 times a week for 30-minutes.*

- *Committed to follow a proven plan that is set in place.*

- *Ready and highly interested in investing in your health now.*

- *Ready to eliminate all of the excuses. This includes, "The diet starts on Monday," because it never does.*

THIS PROGRAM IS NOT FOR YOU IF....

- *If you are looking for another "diet plan." This is NOT for you.*

- *If you want to dabble in a program without putting in the effort.*

- *If you are late for a coaching call and just looking to waste my time.*

- *Refuse to invest in the Bode Pro plan suggested to you.*

- *Refuse to exercise at least 5 times a week for 30-minutes.*

- *Waiting too long to make a decision and need permission to succeed.*

- *Think that this program is a "magic pill." It's not. You actually have to put in the work.*

- Not looking to invest in a coach and complain all day long.

- Not interested at all in anything you have read so far.

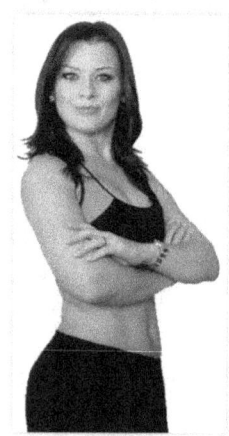

WHAT IS THE NEXT STEP

Now, before you get this program, let me tell you exactly what you get....so that you know it's right for you.

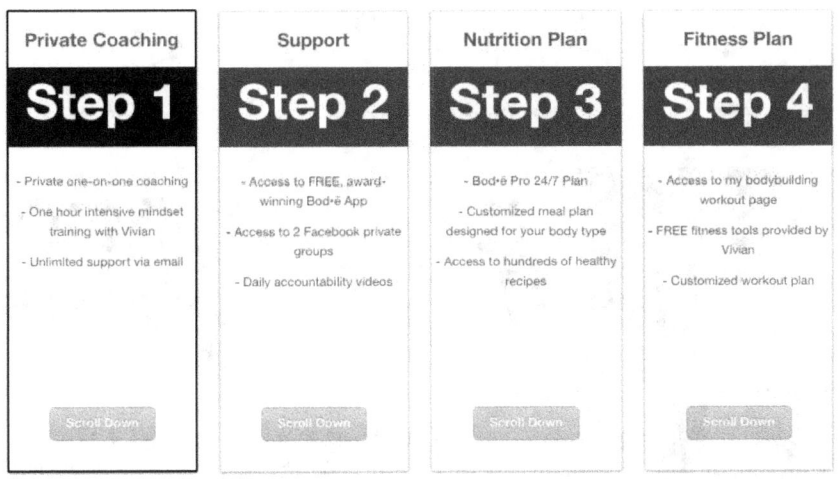

Private Coaching	Support	Nutrition Plan	Fitness Plan
Step 1	**Step 2**	**Step 3**	**Step 4**
- Private one-on-one coaching - One hour intensive mindset training with Vivian - Unlimited support via email	- Access to FREE, award-winning Bod-ë App - Access to 2 Facebook private groups - Daily accountability videos	- Bod-ë Pro 24/7 Plan - Customized meal plan designed for your body type - Access to hundreds of healthy recipes	- Access to my bodybuilding workout page - FREE fitness tools provided by Vivian - Customized workout plan
Scroll Down	Scroll Down	Scroll Down	Scroll Down

GET FIT COACHING PROGRAM

Click <u>here</u> to view my amazing <u>coaching program</u> designed just for you.

LIVE EVENTS

This event is open to female professionals who are ready to take their life to the next level. You know it's time to raise your standards and you are ready to take all out massive action. Join me in Phoenix, AZ on June 9-15 as my team and I host an incredible event just for you!

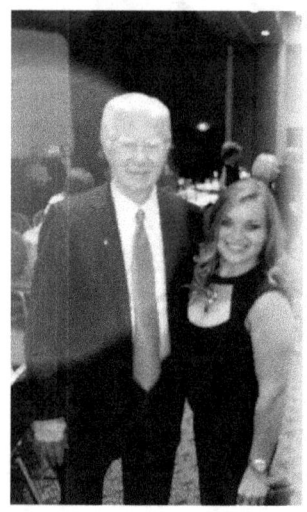

#*lady*BOSS
LEADERSHIP
Training Event

"You're first and foremost job as a LEADER is to take charge of your own energy." - Bob Proctor

When: June 9-15, 2015
Where: Phoenix, AZ

Note: Acceptance to the LadyBoss Leadership Training Event is by application ONLY. Our team will hand select who is eligible to attend. Once accepted, we will contact you to let you know what is your next step.

Click on the button below to start your application. You will be directed to fill out a questionnaire. This will help our team decide if this training event is a good fit for you.

YAY, LETS CONNECT!

"PROVE THAT THE IMPOSSIBLE IS POSSIBLE."
- VIVIAN WEISSMAN

WHO IS VIVIAN WEISSMAN

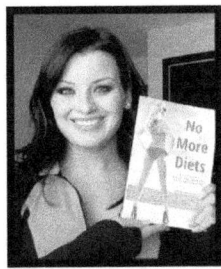

With Bob Proctor

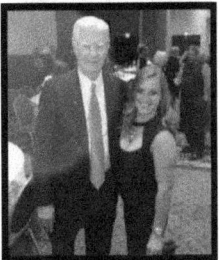

With Darren Hardy

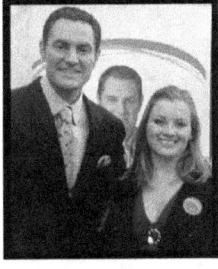

Vivian Weissman is the best selling author of No More Diets and one of the top in-demand trainers in the personal development and fitness industry.

Her purpose has always been to inspire and instruct people how to create their life by design and fully access their unlimited potential. After realizing that it was a blessing to be born at 24 weeks and being paralyzed from the waist down, Vivian freely and openly shares her life's work based on experience on how to create a meaningful, fulfilled and compelling future.

For over a decade, she has dedicated her life to helping individuals, teams, and organizations find their true calling to live a more happy, health and wealthy lifestyle without compromise.

Recognized as a thought leader, Vivian travels all over the world focusing on sharing her unique strategies and philosophies on success, leadership, goal achieving and persistence.

Granted, her clients include non-profit organizations such as Street Partners of Wall Street, entrepreneurs from 50+ countries and female executives looking to massively improve their results in business and life.

HOW CAN VIVIAN WEISSMAN HELP YOU

Are you a super busy female professional who is tired of being sick and tired of getting the same results in fitness and weight loss? Have you been on a million diets too and wondered why it worked for others, but not you? Feeling confused right about now?

I've been in your shoes too many times to count, so I know how you feel. Even though I have been in the fitness industry for over 10 years, I've secretly struggled with an eating disorder and believed that if you look good on the outside then you must be "healthy."

What I have found through personal experience is that the only reason I jumped from one diet to the next is because I was brainwashed by the media to believe it was the only way to lose weight. The real problem was me. My relationship with myself was not healthy and I was obsessed with getting down to a size zero. Measuring everything became a destructive habit.

I know that you have felt the same way. You have also tried those fad diets and felt like it was never the right fit for you for some reason. Deep down you knew going on a "diet" was unhealthy, but you did it anyway.

Here's the thing. What really changed for me was when I invested in myself and found a mentor that showed me that it has nothing to do with what weight management program you're on. It all has to do with your mindset. In order for you to have an amazing life where dieting is no longer the option, you have to work on yourself. Working on you is the starting point. That is the driving force to why you do what you do.

Listen, research is not going to provide you with the results you truly seek that will last. If the *real solution* was doing research and following a "diet plan," then you wouldn't feel stuck, frustrated and confused.

Everyone is different physiologically. One plan is not going to work for another. The good news is, what does work is the combination of the mindset-work with a proven plan that is customized for your body type.

The only way my clients ever seen long lasting results was when they were able to eliminate all of the self-limiting beliefs and stories that no longer serve them. You can either let your excuses stop you from getting the dream body you have always wanted or figure out why your results are the same.

It's really that simple. If you want to lose weight, feel confident about yourself or even challenge yourself to see what you're capable of doing, the mindset work is super important. Without it, you'll just wonder without a real

game plan set in place. When you make a commitment to yourself that you're no longer settling, that's where the magic happens. That's how you're going to get from where you are, to where you truly desire in your fitness and weight loss goals.

If you don't work on your MINDSET, you can forget about your RESULTS.

Click on the audio below to listen to a SPECIAL interview I did on how to get started and how to achieve success. Want to listen to it on your iPod, iPhone or Android? To download, right click and choose "save as."

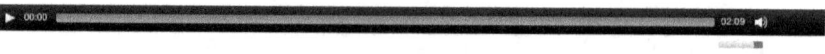

Now, before you invest your time and money, let me tell you exactly what happened and how I transformed my life. This will help you decide if us working together is a good fit for you.

Within a 30 day period, I potentially dropped 30 pounds in 30 days and kept it off for over 3 years. I know a transformation like this can happen for you too. It all comes down to what are you focusing on and what are you committed to? Currently, since I love investing in myself, I have made my own personal commitment to compete at a body building competition in June 2015. I know that your goals are different, but what I am suggesting is for you to raise your standards and find out what you are capable of doing. In the FREE coaching call that I have attached on this page, I share with you why I have decided to achieve this goal.

I know that you are that serious type who loves to gain the support she deserves and wants to be held accountable for her actions. If that is you and you're serious about making a change in your life, I'm willing to commit and work with you so that you achieve the results you are looking for right now.

Look, I've been on yo-yo diets before just like you. I have tried fasting, raw food juice cleansing and even working out at the gym for three hours to lose weight. Nothing was working! I've always felt like a diet was something temporary and that as soon as I lose the weight, then I can go back to how I used to live. Diets do not work. Counting calories and counting points do not work either. And that familiar phrase, "diet starts on Monday" is just an excuse. Lets keep it real.

My focus is to really help you understand why you do what you do so that you develop those strong habits that will lead to your success. Honestly, if you want to lose weight and finally keep it off for good, it has nothing to do with what you eat and going on another one of those "programs." If you are looking for lasting change and really transforming your body, your mindset has to shift.

To be really transparent with you, a few years ago I've neglected my health because of my busy schedule. That enabled me to gain 30 pounds and at that point I really didn't know where to start and I lost all hope. Ironically, I was the top personal trainer in New York, so it would make sense for me to know what to do next and how to lose weight. Right?

When you lose hope of any possibility of getting your dream body back, it's hard to get started and get back to creating positive momentum. That's when I had my aha-moment and realized that it had nothing to do with dieting and exercising. My results are a direct reflection of me and my self image. The real transformation first happened on the inside and with my thinking. It was only a matter of time when my results caught up to me. When I have made a decision to invest in a high level coach and get one-on-one support, that's when the real shift happened. I no longer needed to go on another diet and the excuse of "it's hard to find the time" was out the window.

So, if you're truly committed to giving your absolute best and kicking all of your excuses aside, lets take the first step together and see my Get Fit Coaching Program is right for you. Click here to listen to my 60-minute FREE coaching call to learn more about what I can offer you.

"The power of environment says to be the same because of our deepest desire to have love and connection. Consciously you don't associate food with emotions. Once you replace the emotional addictiveness and detach from the meaning, your intuition tells you what the body needs. That is what Vivian Weissman is teaching." - *Kal Malik, Speaker and Author*

Click on the audio below to listen to a 4-minute interview of how my client virtually lost 38-pounds in less than 6 weeks. Want to listen to it on your iPod, iPhone or Android? To download, right click and choose "save as."

MY RESULTS

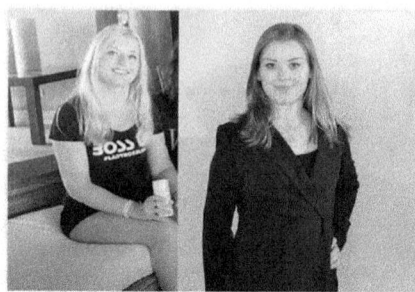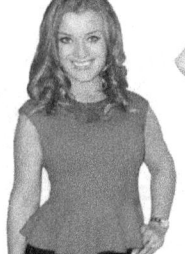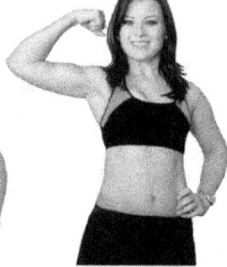

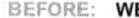

BEFORE: **WEIGHT:** 140 **DRESS SIZE:** 16 **AFTER:** **WEIGHT:** 110 **DRESS SIZE:** 2

GET FIT COACHING PROGRAM

Click here to view my amazing coaching program designed just for you.

How Would You Love To Work With Vivian Weissman Directly?

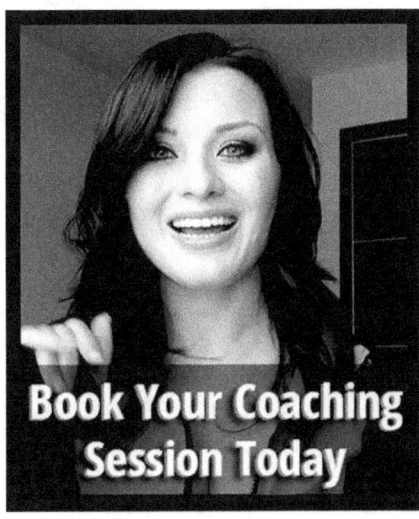

Vivian Weissman is a world-renowned business trainer and fitness coach with more than 12 years experience in the personal development industry.

Recognized as one of the top in-demand trainers, Vivian enables sales team organizations and entrepreneurs find their true passions in life, increase performance and productivity with her proven training programs.

Granted, her clients include non-profit organizations such as Street Partners of Wall Street, business leaders from 50+ countries and female executives looking to massively improve their results in business and life.

If you ever wanted to transform your life and take your results to new levels, then this opportunity is for you!

With this private coaching opportunity, you will be trained personally by me.

Take Action Now To See If You Qualify To Be Apart Of Our

12 Month Intensive Coaching Program.

http://vivianfitness.com/book-session/

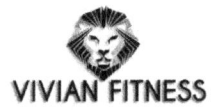

VIVIAN FITNESS